THE DYING PROCESS

YOUR ESSENTIAL GUIDE TO UNDERSTANDING SIGNS, SYMPTOMS & CHANGES AT THE END OF LIFE

KATIE DUNCAN

NURSE PRACTITIONER

CONTENTS

The Crucial Toolkit For End-Of-Life Care	v
Preface	ix
Introduction	xi
1. 1-3 Months Before Death	1
2. 1-3 Weeks Before Death	6
3. Approaching Death	21
4. Hours to Days Before Death	25
5. Minutes Before Death	34
6. How Do I Know When My Loved One Has Died?	36
Conclusion	43
Please Share	47
7. Bonus	49
Acknowledgments	53
About the Author	57
The Crucial Toolkit For End-Of-Life Care	59
References	61

© **Copyright Katie Duncan 2021 - All rights reserved.**

Legal Notice:

This book is copyright protected. This book is only for personal use. The content contained within this book may not be reproduced, duplicated, distributed, sold, used, quoted, paraphrased, or transmitted, in whole or in part, without the direct written consent of the author or the publisher.

Disclaimer Notice:

Under no circumstances will any blame or legal responsibility be held against the publisher, or author, for any damages, reparation, or monetary loss due to the information contained within this book. Either directly or indirectly. You are responsible for your own choices, actions, and results.

The information contained in this book is for personal educational and entertainment purposes only. The content is derived from various sources, and the author has done her best to present accurate, up-to-date, and reliable, complete information. Readers acknowledge the author is not engaging in the rendering of legal, financial, medical, or professional advice. Readers must consult with appropriate licensed professionals before utilizing any of the techniques or approaches described in this book. Under no circumstances will the author be held responsible for any damage or loss incurred as a result of a reader's decision to follow any advice offered herein - even in the event of errors, omission, or inaccuracies - in the absence of, or in contradiction of, independent professional guidance.

THE CRUCIAL TOOLKIT FOR END-OF-LIFE CARE

Get Your Exclusive Copy Now!

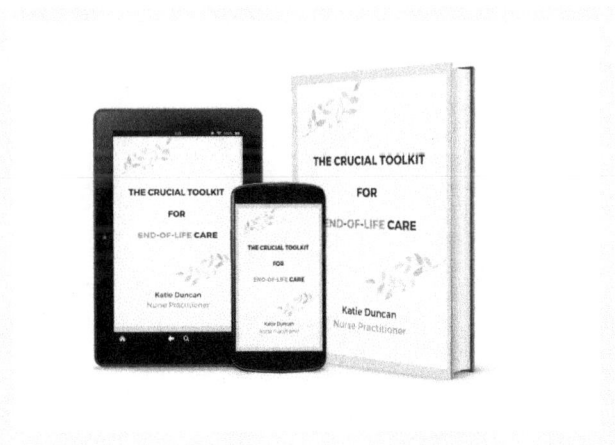

Insert the link below into your browser:
www.deathcarecoach.com

To humanity,
may you be at peace at the end of your journey.

PREFACE

"It is the unknown we fear when we look upon death and darkness, nothing more."

— Albus Dumbledore

INTRODUCTION

"No one wants to die. Even people who want to go to heaven don't want to die to get there. And yet death is the destination we all share. No one has ever escaped it. And that is as it should be, because death is very likely the single best invention of life. It is life's change agent. It clears out the old to make way for the new."

— Steve Jobs

You just found out someone you love is dying.

The rush of emotion bombards you...

Shock.

You're numb.

"No."

"This must be a mistake."

"There must be something we can do."

"No."

"We'll do anything."

"What are our options?"

"We are going to find a cure."

"I'm going to save you."

"You're not going to die."

"He's not going to die."

"She's not going to die."

"They are not going to die."

You slowly begin to settle into this new reality and influx of compounding emotion. Multiple sensations popping up at different moments for any length of time...

They consume you.

It feels suffocating.

Anger. Sadness. Confusion. Helplessness. Anxiety. Overwhelm.

You feel completely lost.

You feel as if you are drowning in pain and heartache.

You ask yourself, "What will I do without them?"

…At some point, you reach some version of acceptance. **Because you have no other choice.**

You realize you must shove your emotions away for now. And quickly. Because *now* you have to figure out how to be a caregiver, how *you* will take care of them, and how *you* will help keep them comfortable during a time that feels anything but.

Yet suddenly, you realize, "I have no idea what dying looks like." And how would you, unless you have seen it before?

You think…

"How do I know what to expect? How do I know what to prepare for? How do I know what to do?"

The impact of emotion hits hard yet again…

Fear. Overwhelm. Pain. Emptiness.

You feel unprepared.

If this is you or someone you know, keep reading. This guide is for you. In your moments of fear, deep sadness, and overwhelm, this is the guide you can turn to for answers. I hope it will empower you.

I have worked in the healthcare profession in various roles for over a decade as a technician, nurse, nurse practitioner, and professor. I have provided patient care in hospital and community settings, as well as assisted living, independent living, nursing home and rehabilitation facilities. For many years, I also provided in-home end-of-life hospice care.

I have had the honor of being at the bedside of many of my precious fellow humans as they approached and eventually took their last breaths in this physical world. And I have been graced with the opportunity to be with their families and loved ones as they worked through these difficult and painful times. I have watched as they somehow found courage and strength through their grief.

Having been present in these moments, I have realized, both professionally and personally, that much of western society has an overarching sense of fear and distress of death and dying. We learn to see death and dying as a tragic failure, which it is not. Rather, it is simply a part of our life's journey. It is a part of our story.

Dying is very much a part of living. And death is a natural part of all of our lives. With every life comes death. This is what makes us human. As hard as we try, we cannot escape it. While we hate to acknowledge it, and as much as we try to hide from it, we are all, in fact, mortal beings. And it is our mortality that makes our lives **precious, treasured,** and **meaningful**.

We don't like to talk about death in Western society, and we generally avoid talking about dying. It's taboo. It's sad. And it's uncomfortable. So instead, we run from it. We hide from it. We avoid talking about it and thinking about it at all costs. The problem with not talking about death and dying is that now we have no idea what to say, what to do, or how to act when this inevitable part of our lives approaches, whether for ourselves or for someone we love.

Generally speaking, even medical professionals are uncomfortable talking about death and dying. In healthcare, we are taught to fix. We are taught to cure. We are taught to save lives. So even we don't like to admit, believe, or even recognize when someone is dying. We feel we must offer a "treatment option" even if that treatment is one that may take away the quality of someone's life. Society leads us all, even many healthcare professionals, to believe end-of-life care is giving up on life.

Unfortunately, because of this, end-of-life care is not frequently offered as a treatment option, even when it may be the most important and best treatment there is. When end-of-life care is recommended, healthcare providers often wait until it's too late, leaving families lost, overwhelmed, and unprepared to care for their dying loved one with their death too quickly approaching.

Throughout most of my life, I have had a curious interest in human life. The entire experience, from birth to death, the process of living in between, and whatever just might exist beyond. The human experience simply *fascinates* me.

I first witnessed death and dying as a young child when my family stood in the veterinarian's office as we watched our dog, Sandy, be put down after a long and hard battle with cancer. I watched as she closed her eyes and went to sleep so peacefully. I remember feeling sad but relieved that she could finally be at peace, her memories forever with me.

I later witnessed death and dying as a teenager when my grandfather suffered a sudden brain aneurysm. Though I wasn't at his bedside when he died, I had seen him go from life to life-support and agreed as our family came to that decision. Later, as a healthcare technician and an intensive care unit nurse, I witnessed death in the hospital setting. Similar to my grandfather, death occurred mainly from critical illness or following the removal of life support.

Despite my many encounters with death, I must be totally honest: It wasn't until I began my journey as a hospice nurse that I became captivated by the death and dying process of us humans. It wasn't until I stood at the bedside, watching as human existence beautifully and uniquely transitioned from life to death - from here in our physical realm to somewhere beyond my eyes' sight - that I fully came to appreciate life as an extraordinary journey from birth *through* death, from beginning to end, and maybe, beyond.

What I have come to realize is that there are many similarities between birth and death. We know and understand that birth is a process. To come into this world, it takes transitions; it takes labor; it takes time. Some births are fast, and some are slow. Some are emergencies, and some happen smoothly. Some are more painful, others less so. Some occur in the middle of the night, some in the middle of the day. Some are alone, and some are surrounded by others. Every birth is messy. Every birth is unique. Every birth has a way of being beautiful.

Death and dying are just the same. Dying is a process consisting of transitions. Death is the final transition. Sometimes it is sudden, and sometimes it is gradual. Some may experience pain, while others may feel no pain at all. Some are messy; others are quite calm. Some die alone, while others die surrounded by loved ones. Dying is intimate, personal, and the most vulnerable part of our lives. It can occur any time, any day. Death and dying are unique. And like birth, death and dying can also be one of the most beautiful experiences we will face in this adventure we call life.

Keep in mind that every person's end-of-life journey is different. This guidebook discusses the process of dying slowly due to age or disease, for example. Some will display all of the signs and symptoms discussed here in this book, while others may experience very few.

Similarly, the timeframes I describe are not set in stone. While I have witnessed many death and dying experiences to make general estimates of remaining lifetime, that is exactly what they are. These are "guesstimates." It is impossible to know exactly when someone will die. So please give yourself permission to be patient with their process, finding presence and gratitude for each day you have them.

I firmly believe that being given the treatment option of "end-of-life care" or "hospice care" is a gift, a priceless gift of time. Time that allows us to be present with our loved one in the final stages of their life story. Time for any last words, thoughts, or wishes to be exchanged.

I will try in this book to give you some tools and guidance to allow you, your family, and others to appreciate the opportunity you have to share the end-of-life, death and dying experience with your loved one. I hope that this guidebook will help calm your mind, prepare you for what to expect as your loved one nears death, and offer some suggestions for simple ways you can help comfort your loved one throughout their dying process.

Your loved one deserves to die in peace, and you deserve *not* to feel helpless or alone. I hope this guidebook will help you achieve <u>both</u> of these important goals.

Before you begin this read, I leave you with my personal perspective on death and dying…

Dying is like the sunset at the end of each day as it beautifully transforms and uniquely lights up the sky even after the sun is no longer in sight...

— KATIE DUNCAN

1

1-3 MONTHS BEFORE DEATH

"To the well-organized mind, death is nothing but the next great adventure."

— J.K. Rowling

D*isconnect*
In the months leading up to death, your loved one will likely begin to disconnect from the world in both small and more noticeable ways. Please know that the following signs and symptoms are a normal part of the dying process. This disconnecting process is your loved one's mind, body, and spirit beginning to slow down in preparation for death.

Sleep is the primary way our bodies find rest and is also one of the earliest signs of withdrawal you are likely to see. For example, you may notice your loved one sleeping more than usual. They may be waking up later and later each morning. They may nap or doze off during the daytime. They may be off to bed for the night earlier and earlier.

Sleep allows your loved one to recover and regain energy for the periods of time they are awake, to be more present with you. You do not need to wake them. Allow them to sleep, help them to bed, cover them with a blanket, tuck them in and kiss them goodnight. Remember sleep is the body and mind's space to rest peacefully. So let them sleep. They may just be dreaming about something special.

When your loved one is awake, they will often seem less and less interested in their everyday life and the world around them. They may stop turning on the morning news. They may stop watching their favorite sports. They may stop asking questions about other people or events. They may not be talkative or have many conversations with you.

Your loved one can appear to be **disengaged**. You may notice they are more **forgetful**, and you may have to remind them of simple things, especially short-term memories. It may seem like they don't care, but please don't be hurt by this. They are not pulling away consciously or on purpose. Your loved one's mind is beginning to naturally detach from the world around them as they prepare to leave it.

. . .

Decreased Appetite

Similarly, your loved one's desire for **food** and water may become less and less. One day their appetite may be normal; the next, they may have none at all. **Weight-loss** is expected.

Keep in mind that when your loved one is dying, their body's physical needs are changing. Your loved one is at the point in their life's journey where their body is beginning to slow down and shut down, and therefore, food and water are no longer their body's physical priority or need. As a result, your loved one may not feel hungry.

They may deny you or refuse when you ask them to eat. As their family member, friend or caregiver, I know this can feel scary. It feels hard to accept because you think your loved one *needs* to eat. Your fears may lead you to wonder,

"Should we start artificial feeding?"

Forcing nutrition on your loved one's body is *not beneficial* when this is <u>not</u> what their body wants or needs. Doing so can even be harmful.

Abdominal discomfort, nausea, vomiting, diarrhea, and choking or reflux that can lead to pneumonia, breathing complications, and even sudden death are just a few of those serious risks.

Help your loved one by allowing *them* to guide *you*. This is especially true with respect to food and water. You do not need to force, and you do not always need to ask.

Instead, let your loved one tell you *if* and *when* they would like something to eat. You may give them what they ask for, even if you feel it is an "unhealthy" option. Providing their requests will give them back some control, **empowering** them in the last days of their life.

Decreased Energy

Slowly, you will begin to notice your loved one is not as active as they once were. They're not going outside as often. They're not going to events. They're not exercising. They're not even moving as much throughout their home. Both their **energy** level and their **muscle** strength are slowly beginning to fade.

When you notice your loved one becoming weaker, ask your healthcare team about recommended **assistive devices** to keep them safe while supporting their mobility for as long as possible. Equipment such as a cane, a walker, a wheelchair, a bedside commode, a Hoyer-lift, and even a hospital bed may help keep your loved one secure.

In addition, you may begin to assist them as they relocate, or move from their bed to a chair. If only for minimal support, offer your arm for your loved one to hold. For more stability, hold onto the waistband of their pants.

2

1-3 WEEKS BEFORE DEATH

"Our death is not an end if we can live on in our children and the younger generation. For they are us; our bodies are only wilted leaves on the tree of life."

— Albert Einstein

During the last month, you've noticed an **ongoing gradual decline** in your loved one. In the weeks leading up to death, your loved one's body will slow down and shut down even further. The disconnecting and disengaging processes will become more obvious and more pronounced.

Your loved one will be sleeping more and more until they are **sleeping** most of every single day. They are likely to appear more and more distant and **withdrawn**. They will have little to say and may not appear to be aware of their surroundings. They may **stare off** into the distance as if they are in a daze.

Their appetite and fluid intake will continue to dwindle to a minimum. Weight-loss will be more obvious now as the bones of their temples, eyelids, cheeks, clavicles, ribs, and maybe hips begin to protrude. This is called **cachexia**.

A *gitation*

Your loved one may start to have periods of **restlessness**, agitation, **delirium**, or **confusion**. They may tug at their clothes or blankets, yell or call out, speak nonsensically, or be unaware of who you are or where they are. You may notice this happening repeatedly at certain times of the day, especially in the afternoon or evening. This is called **sundowning**.

The most supportive thing you can do at this time is to remain calm. You can try to reorient your loved one to their surroundings. Remind them of who they are, where they are, and who you are. Remind them they are *safe.*

Other soothing techniques such as dimming bright lights, playing soft **music**, spraying lavender scents in the room, or gently rubbing their arm and holding their hand may be helpful.

You know your loved one best. What do they typically do for relaxation? Try these things.

Your healthcare team may suggest anti-anxiety medications such as Lorazepam or antipsychotic medications such as Haloperidol, which may also help your loved one remain calm. However, it's important to note, in some cases, these medications may intensify agitation. You and your healthcare team will work together to find a balance between medication and non-medication techniques to manage it effectively.

Hallucinations

It is common to have vision-like experiences or **hallucinations** at the end of life. Your loved one may tell you they are seeing people or pets that have died before them. They may see other visitors who are unfamiliar. Your loved one may even have conversations with these visitors or hear them speaking.

Regardless of your own beliefs, understand that these visions are very real to your loved one. Rather than deny their visions, be **curious** and acknowledge them. Ask your loved one to describe who they are seeing and what these visitors are saying. If your loved one appears scared, again remind them they are safe.

I once met an older woman with dementia in the last months of her life. When I met her, she had not been verbal for several years. As she neared her final days, her husband and I both noticed her constant gaze toward the left corner of her bedroom.

One afternoon, while staring into that same left corner of the room, the woman spoke. With her husband at her side, she said to him,

---

"Your mother is here with me."

That was all. Two days later, she died. Her husband and I both believed she went with his mother when she took her last breaths.

Before bringing him home on hospice care, my Granddad had been in and out of the hospital on multiple occasions. In the days leading up to his final discharge home, my Granddad had only brief moments of energy and few moments of complete lucidity.

Almost every time he opened his eyes, I began to notice he would instinctively stare upwards and slightly off to the right, just beyond the clock on the wall in front of him. I knew what was happening. He was seeing someone or something unseen to me.

One evening, he called me over to his bedside. I asked if he was alright and reinforced that I was here with him. He whispered to me softly,

> "I need you to know I'm not totally here. I need you to know they keep coming to see me."

I attempted to question him further, but his response remained,

> "You know."

Then he squeezed my hand and closed his eyes.

With my years of end-of-life work and our shared stories of my experiences, he knew that I knew. And I did. I knew whoever he was seeing would guide him wherever he went when he left this world.

These are only two of many stories I could share with you; incredible stories some of you may not even believe. I have witnessed so many amazing experiences throughout others' end-of-life journeys that I am no longer surprised to hear of strange, unusual, and unimaginable happenings as death approaches.

Abdominal Issues

Your loved one's appetite will almost certainly continue to decline. They will not eat or drink much if anything at all. They may also have a more difficult time **chewing** and **swallowing**. Soft foods such as pudding or applesauce may be easier to manage as they do not require chewing. Additionally, shakes or smoothies are thick, tasty, and may be easier to swallow.

You may notice their **mouth** and **lips** becoming quite dry. Continue to help your loved one keep their mouth clean. We all know the feeling of a freshly cleaned mouth after brushing our teeth. Yet, it is a daily comfort that we often don't think much about. Not only does a clean mouth *feel* good, but it also lowers the risk of your loved one developing an infection.

Ask your healthcare team about **mouth swabs** (small sponge on a stick) to help clean and moisten your loved one's teeth, gums, and tongue.

Dip the mouth swab in liquid such as, water, gatorade, or alcohol-free mouthwash. Then, gently dab the mouth swab on the side of the cup to remove excess liquid. This will help prevent unwanted liquid from dripping down the back of your loved one's throat. The mouth swab should be just slightly moist. Softly and quickly brush the mouth swab against your loved one's teeth, tongue, cheeks, gums, and lips.

If you notice your loved one begin to unconsciously bite down on these swabs, please be cautious. It can be difficult to remove anything from their reflexive bite. The more you pull, the harder they may clench. Instead, try gently rubbing underneath their chin, cheek, or elsewhere to relax their jaw.

When your loved one is alert, you can assist them with brushing their teeth or rinsing their mouth. Avoid alcohol-based mouthwash as this may worsen their dryness. **Ice-chips** and **popsicles** may also provide relief. But as before, do not try to force them to eat or drink if they do not want to. Doing so may lead to complications mentioned previously.

If your loved one is using oxygen therapy, <u>avoid</u> petroleum-based products such as Vaseline to moisten their lips/nose/face. Instead, <u>use</u> **water-based** products such as Aloe Vera or K-Y jelly.

Nausea and **vomiting** episodes are quite common experiences at the end of life. One cause may be related to the chemical and hormonal changes within the body, which may lead to overstimulation of the body's vomiting response. Nausea may also be caused by constipation or blockage somewhere within your loved one's digestive tract. Additionally, food becomes more difficult to tolerate as your loved one's digestive tract continues to slow.

Depending on your loved one's situation, their healthcare provider may provide several recommendations to help treat their nausea. For example, they may advise avoiding food and fluid for a period of time to allow the digestive tract to rest. Once nausea has improved, they may suggest small sips of clear liquids such as water, broth, jello, or tea, followed by bland foods such as crackers or toast.

Your healthcare provider may also prescribe medications to help treat nausea, such as Ondansetron or Haloperidol.

Your loved one will be moving their bowels and urinating less often. They may even begin to lose control of their **urination** and **bowel movements** altogether, with minimal or no awareness. This is called **incontinence**.

At this stage, you may find it helpful to use **disposable briefs** such as diapers or pull-ups, as well as washable/disposable **underpads** that can be placed flat underneath your loved one's hips while in bed. Like the wet doggy pads you might use for puppy training, these will help to absorb leaky urine. You will find this beneficial as your loved one may not be able to get out of bed or reach the bathroom quickly or safely anymore.

In addition, your healthcare team might suggest a **foley catheter** - a tube placed into the bladder to direct their urine to a collection bag – to cut down the chances that moisture and urine will irritate their skin. It may also help decrease painful movements by reducing the number of times you will need to change their undergarments.

Weakness

Your loved one's **muscles** will continue to weaken, eventually needing assistance moving themselves in bed. Hospital beds allow for easy repositioning using remote-controlled adjustments for both the upper and lower body, helping to keep your loved one safe and comfortable.

When your loved one cannot move around in bed any longer, continue to **reposition** them to avoid lying in one position for too long. For example, place **pillows** underneath the length of their back and hip to turn your loved one slightly off to one side. You can also set a pillow between their knees. Then, two hours later, switch the pillows to roll them slightly to the opposite side.

At first, it can be challenging to reposition your loved one by yourself, so if possible, it may be helpful to have someone else to assist. If you are the sole caretaker, ask your healthcare team to show you tips on how to reposition your loved one.

Skin

You will notice changes to your loved one's skin. Their **skin** will become thin, **fragile**, and easily prone to tears, bruising, or injury. Typical areas of skin breakdown are the buttocks, hips, and heals due to the constant pressure placed upon them.

To protect their skin and comfort their joints, place pillows underneath their elbows, hips, wrists, knees, and heals. You can also use pillows to help turn, reposition, and support your loved one's joints and skin.

While these simple techniques may lower the risk of skin breakdown, bedsores are often unavoidable as your loved one's body continues to shut down. Your healthcare team may suggest the application of different skin protectant **lotions, balms,** or **patches** for added protection.

. . .

Pain

For most of us, our primary concern is…

"How will I keep my loved one **pain-free**?"

In the last several weeks of life, there is a possibility of pain. However, some will experience no pain at all.

Pain at the end of life is complex. *Pain* is subjective, meaning each of us perceives and feels pain differently.

Some pain is physical. Some pain is emotional. Some pain is psychological. Sometimes, emotional and psychological distress manifests as physical pain.

Some people may have pain as they near death due to their specific illness(es).

There are many **pain-relief** treatment options available. Your loved one's pain-type will dictate the best pain management techniques for the most pain control.

Your healthcare team may have specific medication recommendations depending on pain-type. Therefore, it is always a good idea to let your healthcare team know if your loved one is, or seems to be, experiencing any type of pain.

Medications such as **Morphine** or other opioids are common end-of-life pain treatments.

Societal concerns about these medications may cause worry that Morphine will speed up your loved one's death or lead to an addiction.

However, uncontrolled pain may be more likely to speed up the dying process due to the stress pain puts on the body. In addition, these medications are for short-term use specifically to manage end of life pain, and therefore worries regarding addiction are not of concern.

Managing your loved one's pain as they approach death is the top priority as this is a significant contributor to the **quality** of their life. Morphine or similar medications are often the most effective medications for doing so.

Pain medications and doses are **safely** adjusted based on the type of pain your loved one is experiencing.

It is much easier to **prevent pain** altogether than to relieve pain your loved one is already experiencing, especially if that pain is severe. Therefore, it is crucial to give your loved one pain medications **around the clock** at scheduled times exactly as your healthcare team prescribes, rather than medicating as their pain worsens.

If your loved one's pain becomes uncontrolled, your healthcare team may adjust medications and doses as needed.

You may also be able to provide pain relief without the use of medications. For example, simply repositioning your loved one on their side or lifting them higher in bed may relieve body ache or tension.

Similarly, **heating pads** or **ice packs** (covered by a towel) for twenty minutes at a time may help with muscle or joint aches.

You might also try alternative soothing techniques, focusing on your loved one's **five senses**: seeing, hearing, smelling, tasting, and feeling.

For example, try **dimming** bright lights or placing **photos** of loved ones near the bed. Play their favorite **music** softly or hum their favorite lullaby. Light **candles** with their favorite smell. Aromatherapy such as **lavender** scented oils or sprays also shows to have calming effects. Dip mouth swabs in their favorite drinks to give them a small taste of the **flavor** on their tongue. Finally, a gentle arm, leg, foot, shoulder, or back-rub (or **massage**) with their favorite lotion may relieve pain sensations and provide comfort.

If your loved one is more alert, slow gentle **breathing** and **meditation** may relax their mind and body.

Using this Opportunity

These changes in behavior and body function can come on quite suddenly. It can easily alarm you and send red flag signals to your brain. Rather than allowing these alerts to increase your anxiety, recognize them as a message from your loved one: that they could use your help.

This is your opportunity to be a creative caregiver, finding new and personalized ways of bringing peace to your loved one, deepening your connection with them.

This is yet another **rewarding gift** of time: the time to reach out to anyone your loved one may want to see while they are still somewhat awake and alert, for example.

It is also a time to **communicate** with them while they are still conscious, even if their response is minimal. If you feel lost for words, try sitting with a pen and paper in hand. Write your loved one a **letter**.

When my Granddad was dying, I couldn't seem to find my words. So this is exactly what I did. I wrote a letter, my thoughts flowing onto that piece of paper when only minutes before my mind had felt numb. I had been hesitant to read him my letter because he had been minimally alert. I wasn't sure he would hear me, or understand me. But, I did. Reading that letter to him, and hearing his simple response,

---

"And *I* love you,"

gave me closure. It gave me peace of mind and heart.

Hearing is thought to be the last sense to leave us when we are dying.

So, read your loved one your letter. They can hear you, even if they can't respond.

The words you share with your loved one might be a simple "Thank you" or "I love you" or "I will miss you" or maybe even "I forgive you." Grant them the comfort of your peace, your grace, and your love.

3

APPROACHING DEATH

"The most basic and powerful way to connect to another person is to listen. Just listen. Perhaps the most important thing we ever give each other is our attention.... A loving silence often has far more power to heal and to connect than the most well-intentioned words."

— RACHEL NAOMI REMEN

As the death of your loved one approaches, your focus will (and should) likely be on offering the kinds of comfort and support I've discussed in the previous chapters. At the same time, you will be finding ways to cope with your own grief and that of others you love.

In this chapter, I've identified things that will be beneficial to think about *before* your loved one dies. While your energy is likely running thin, I encourage you to set a time to organize these important tasks.

Appoint A Spokesperson

As the caregiver for a dying loved one, it seems friends, family, and others expect you to give constant updates. The phone keeps ringing. New texts and emails appear daily. Quite honestly, it can be exhausting. As it is, your mind, body, and soul are trying to keep up one day at a time. Grant yourself permission to protect your energy. You and your loved one deserve this.

To help prevent burnout, delegate a spokesperson, someone who will communicate to others on your behalf and the only person you will need to keep informed. This person may be a close friend, another family member, or someone you trust. Feel encouraged to **direct** everyone to this dedicated spokesperson from the start of your loved one's end-of-life journey. Release the pressure of this responsibility.

Finances

You will want to know of and have access to all of your loved one's **finances** and **assets**. This includes, but is not limited to, trust funds, personal property, bank accounts, investments, retirement accounts, safety deposit boxes, insurance policies, bill payments, and any others.

Accounts

After your loved one dies, you will need to access or close accounts and **notify** several **agencies** of your loved one's death. This will likely include some or all of the following: banks or other financial institutions, life insurance companies, the social security administration, financial advisors or stockbrokers, personal or estate lawyers, accountants, credit card agencies, the department of motor vehicles, insurance agencies, etc.

You may also want to think about closing and deleting or managing **email** accounts and **social media** accounts.

Funeral Home Decisions

Lastly, funeral home personnel often play a vital role after the death of your loved one. Because of this, it is helpful to have made some key decisions about the funeral home *before* your loved one dies.

Selecting a funeral home **in advance** is essential because it is unlikely you will have the emotional capacity to easily make decisions the moment of their death.

Think about whether your loved one will be buried or cremated. Think about where you may want to lay their body or ashes.

Your loved one may very well have already prepared these arrangements for themselves. They may have already contacted and paid for the funeral home, their casket, and other arrangements.

I recommend calling several different funeral homes to ask **questions** about services offered, prices of those services, and even ask to speak to the **director**. You may find prices vary widely.

It may also be comforting to get to know the director, so you feel confident your loved one will be in compassionate hands. Once you have decided, notify the funeral home of choice to help them prepare and put yourself at ease.

4

HOURS TO DAYS BEFORE DEATH

"Death must be so beautiful. To lie in the soft brown earth, with the grasses waving above one's head, and listen to silence. To have no yesterday, and no tomorrow. To forget time, to forget life, to be at peace."

— OSCAR WILDE

Energy Surge

In the hours to days before your loved one dies, your loved one will have few moments of being awake, alert, and lucid. However, sometimes, you may witness your loved one experience a spontaneous **surge of energy** where they become mentally sharp, lively, participating in spirited conversations, laughing, and maybe even asking for food.

They often request their favorite foods, as if it is their last meal (as it may very well be). Do not be surprised if they only take a bite to enjoy the flavor, soaking it in one last time.

This relatively common energetic time is called **rallying** or a **rally period**. This rally period can last any length of time, from minutes or hours, maybe even an entire day. After what will likely be their final burst of energy, your loved one will sleep deeply, unable to be aroused easily or at all.

I once knew a family who had been sitting vigil by their father's bed for over a week. He hadn't been rousable whatsoever. It seemed everyone was waiting for his final breath.

Then, one morning, he opened his eyes. He told his daughter to invite all the family over *that* day. His daughter, startled as she was, did just that.

They threw him a party. He ate his favorite Italian foods. He laughed. He smiled. He was joking around like nothing was wrong.

After everyone had left, his daughter went to him to say goodnight.

The man simply responded,

"Thank you. Goodnight… I won't be seeing you tomorrow."

She woke the next day and found he had finally taken his last breath.

Eyes

Your loved one's **eyes** will appear glassy, **glazed**, and distant. Their eyelids may stay partially open, and they may stop making eye contact. Both **tearing** and crusts along the eyelids are expected. You can wipe tears and crusts away gently with a tissue or soft, moist towel.

Terminal Agitation

In your loved one's final days, you may notice they become more **restless** and fidgety. This is called **terminal agitation**. They may claw at the air, bedsheets, or clothes. They may appear to be in pain, displaying changes in their facial expressions or experiencing loud outbursts of words, moans, or other noises.

Terminal agitation can occur for many reasons, from physical changes inside the body to emotional changes that can no longer be communicated. It's important to recognize your loved one's behaviors may not necessarily be associated with pain or discomfort and may sometimes be related to adverse medication reactions.

Despite this, as the caregiver, it can be distressing for us to see. The most important thing you can do is remain **calm**, **speak softly** and clearly, and create a **loving** environment for them.

Now is also an excellent time to incorporate simple actions previously mentioned to create a peaceful space. This includes dimming bright lights, lighting candles, playing soft music, adding lavender-scented essential oil aromas, surrounding them with **photos** of family and friends, and gently holding their hands to reassure their safety.

Remember that **energy** is **contagious.** Your calm and peaceful energy may bring your loved one comfort. While fearful and anxious energy may worsen agitation.

Make sure to communicate with your healthcare team as they may recommend or prescribe certain medications to ease pain (like Morphine) or anxiety (like Lorazepam or Haloperidol).

However, sometimes terminal agitation may occur due to excessive use of these medications, so you and your healthcare team will find the **balance** between medication use and the holistic measures mentioned earlier.

Breathing Changes

You will notice changes in your loved one's **breathing patterns** as they near death. Their breathing may at times look very slow, deep, heavy, or even labored. It is also possible to see periods of shallow, faint, or fast breaths.

In addition, you may begin to notice long pauses in between each breath. This is called **apnea.**

As your loved one's body nears death, their breathing function is preparing to stop, which may lead you to believe they are struggling. Please understand these are natural and normal end-of-life transitions.

Your healthcare team may discuss using medications such as **Morphine, inhalers,** or **oxygen** therapy if your loved one appears to be in distress.

Non-medication relief measures can also be effective. For example, sitting your loved one in a **seated** upright position in bed while keeping their **neck** in a neutral (aligned) position will help your loved one breathe more easily.

Sometimes simple things like opening a **window, air conditioning** the room, or turning on a **fan** or a **vaporizer** can be just the trick.

For those who are more alert, **meditation** or slow controlled **breathing** exercises may also be helpful.

Congestion

Along with breathing changes, you may start to hear a sound in the back of your loved one's **throat** similar to **congestion**. This is called a **rattle**. You may notice a wet cough or hear a gurgling sound with each breath.

As caregivers, the congestion and noise can be distressing. While you may believe your loved one is suffering or in pain, they are not. This is a natural part of the body's shutting down process and your loved one is no longer in a fully conscious state of mind. Therefore, researchers believe your loved one is **not** experiencing any **distress**.

Although current evidence shows there is little we can do to improve this congestion, there may be some actions to try. One step that may improve this rattle is to **gently turn** your loved one to **one side** while keeping them in an **upright seated position**.

You can also ask your healthcare team about medications, such as **Hyoscyamine** or **Atropine**, which may help dry the congestion.

If your loved one is having brief moments of consciousness, the congestion may be due to their particular illness(es).

Consider asking your hospice nurse about increasing the use of **Morphine** for comfort sedation.

Temperature Changes

Fevers are likely to develop at the end of life. To decrease your loved one's fever, try bathing your loved one or washing their skin gently with a **cool washrag**. Be sure to pat their skin dry afterward.

Similarly, placing a cool, moist washcloth over their **forehead** for several minutes at a time may be helpful. In addition, cooling the room with **air** conditioning or a **fan** may feel refreshing.

Lastly, your healthcare team may advise medications such as **Acetaminophen** or **Tylenol** in suppository forms that you may administer as prescribed.

Skin

Skin coloring and temperature will continue to change. Depending on your loved one's normal skin tone, you will notice changes, especially to their feet, legs, and hands (furthest away from their heart). Your loved one's skin may feel **cool** and may turn **pale, blue, purple,** or **blotchy** in appearance. As their body is shutting down, blood flow decreases, contributing to these skin changes.

. . .

Giving Permission

During these final hours and days, I cannot stress enough how *important* it is that you give your loved one **permission** to die. Many times, our loved ones will continue to hold onto life, even in an unconscious state, for the sake of those they love. This can cause them more distress. If they fear you are not ready for them to leave you, they might attempt to keep their body alive despite it being prepared to stop.

So tell them to **"*let go*"** whenever they are ready. Of course, you will miss them, and you will be sad. Still, let them know you will recover and be okay. Tell them their family will survive, move forward, and continue their legacy.

Giving your loved one your permission to die is perhaps the **most beautiful gift** you could ever give them. Treasure this knowledge deep in your heart as you permit them to leave this physical world, and launch them with **love** and **grace** into the realms of the unknown.

Offering Space

For reasons we will never be able to explain, our loved ones will not always die when we expect them to. So if, after having said your goodbyes and gifting them permission to die, you are still unsure why your loved one has not let go, you may want to give them more **space** to be alone.

Remember, they are on their journey, not yours. While you may want to be with your loved one when they die, *they* may not want *you* there. It is often in the brief minutes, even seconds, that we leave their room or are not paying attention that they decide to leave this world.

Your loved one may interpret you being present at their bedside to mean you are not ready to lose them despite having said so. Offer space by **leaving their bedside** for some time. With your physical presence no longer right next to them, your loved one may take comfort knowing you will be okay without them.

Turn soft music on, dim the lights, carry out any **religious**, **spiritual**, **cultural**, or **family traditions** you may follow, and then provide them space to leave their bodies and this world in peace.

5
MINUTES BEFORE DEATH

"Death leaves a heartache no one can heal, love leaves a memory no one can steal."

— RICHARD PUZ

In the final minutes before death, your loved one will not be awake or alert. Their **eyes** will appear glossy and may be partially open. Each **breath** will suddenly become shallow, airy, almost **gasp-like**.

If you are at your loved one's side when this time comes, yes, you may hold their hands. Yes, you may **kiss** them. Yes, you may tell them, "Goodbye," "I love you," "It's okay," "We will all be okay," "You can go," or even suggest that they might,

> "Take the hand of [someone special who has died before them] and go with them."

Do not be afraid. Instead, find gratitude for having been given the grace to guide, comfort, and accompany your loved one into this final transition of life into death. As you remain calm, you can begin to notice the **remarkable** and **inescapable** part of human life that death is.

Experience these last invaluable seconds or minutes as you propel your loved one's soul into the unknown with love.

6

HOW DO I KNOW WHEN MY LOVED ONE HAS DIED?

"What we have once enjoyed we can never lose. All that we love deeply becomes a part of us."

— HELEN KELLER

Some of you will be with your loved one as their heart and lungs finally come to a complete stop. Some of you will not.

Some of you will have the opportunity to watch as their spirit moves from their body into a space unrevealed to us. Again, some of you will not.

But, whether you are present or whether you are not, their timing is exactly as it was meant to be.

You will know that your loved one has died when you feel for a pulse on one side of their neck or the thumb side of their inner wrist and no longer feel the tap of their **heartbeat**.

You will no longer see or hear your loved one **breathing**.

Their **eyes** may stay slightly open, and their **jaw** relaxed. Their **body** will be lying still.

Often, you will see the wrinkles and lines on your loved one's face soften as if all their stress has disappeared.

Their **skin** coloring will fade and become cool to the touch.

Still, you may not know for certain whether your loved one has died. In this moment of uncertainty, it's easy to find yourself in a state of panic.

"Are they gone?!" "Is that it?!" "Are they dead?!"

Others of you may have no doubt your loved one has died. But, even in this knowing, you too, may feel frantic.

"They're dead!" "What do I do?!"

In both of these situations, panic, fear, and sadness can easily take over. You knew your loved one would die. You tried to prepare yourself for their death.

Even so, as prepared as you believe you are, you can never be fully ready for the **shock** and **magnitude** of that moment.

As humans, we are instinctively in *"go, go, go"* mode, especially when under enormous distress. And so, you may impulsively and urgently reach for the phone to call your healthcare team, hospice team, or 911.

But, please, **I urge you to wait**...

Instead, <u>do nothing</u>. Simply pause. Take a deep breath. Find stillness. Give yourself permission to be present. Right here. Right now. Beside your loved one. Tune in to the space around you.

Feel the gravity of it all.

It was only seconds or minutes ago that your loved one transitioned out of their body and into the undiscovered. There is an **honor** in being at their bedside and a **privilege** to be within this **divine** space. Find **wonder** in the possibility of their new world- a world we cannot see, hear, taste, smell, or touch. Embrace the **beauty** and **awe** this space offers. **Cherish** it. Do not rush it. You will not get it back.

In this **serenity**, continue to tap into your body, mind, and soul. Allow yourself to connect to the *now*.

> What is taking place within you? What feelings are surfacing? What might be happening with your loved one's soul?

Release any judgment you place on your answers. Acknowledging your feelings allows all parts of you to adjust to this momentous event. You are **re-calibrating** and **re-aligning**. Finding that steadiness will ground you as you make your way through the "after death" to-do's.

Whenever you are ready, anywhere from 5 to 20 minutes later, begin to move <u>*very*</u> slowly. You may now **call** on someone.

Depending on what healthcare team you are working with, call to let them know you believe your loved one has died. They will then work with you on the next steps.

For example, if you are working with a hospice team, a nurse will come to your home (or facility) to assess your loved one, confirm they no longer have a pulse, and contact the funeral home.

You can then expect the **funeral home director** and assistants to arrive within a given time frame (typically within an hour depending on location) to pick up your loved one's body.

When the funeral home director and team arrive, I encourage you to **step** into another room while they assist your loved one out of the house. Watching this process can be incredibly upsetting for some.

Instead of standing by the doorway, do something to **remember** and **celebrate** your loved one by how they *lived*.

From personal experience, I would encourage you to consider an activity that the family can focus on during this time to honor your loved one's life.

While he didn't often drink alcohol, my Granddad, Bob Duncan, loved a good old vodka-tonic on special occasions. Knowing this, my family agreed that on the day of his death, as the funeral home director guided him out of the home he and my Grandma had lived in for almost 60 years, we would each pour our own vodka-tonic (or non-vodka-tonic for those who did not drink alcohol) and say a "cheers" and "thanks" to him.

When that moment arrived, those of us who happened to be at his house walked into the kitchen together, poured our drinks, clinked our glasses, and each said our "I love you's" and our "thank you's."

Our other family members across the country did the same where they were, alone or with others, at home, at work, or wherever.

In that difficult time, we **shared** our videos and pictures toasting my Grandad's incredible soul. We will be forever grateful for that collective moment of **remembrance** and **celebration**.

Soon after the immediate necessities are taken care of, the funeral director will meet with you to better get to know you and your loved one. Then, they will discuss more details in preparation for any funeral arrangements that may take place.

CONCLUSION

"Death will come, no matter what anyone may think about it. Accept it as a necessity, and pass the thought out of your mind. It must be a necessity, or it would not come to all. Perhaps it is not as bad as it has been pictured.

The entire world is made up of only two things, ENERGY and MATTER. In elementary physics we learn that neither matter nor energy (the only two realities known to man) can be created nor destroyed. Both matter and energy can be transformed, but neither can be destroyed. Life is energy, if it is anything.

If neither energy nor matter can be destroyed, of course life cannot be destroyed. Life, like other forms of energy, may be passed through various processes of transition, or change, but it cannot be destroyed. Death is mere transition.

If death is not mere change, or transition, then nothing comes after death except a long, eternal, peaceful sleep, and sleep is nothing to be feared. Thus you may wipe out, forever, the fear of Death."

— Napoleon Hill

As strange, sad, painful, and sometimes unfair as death may seem, it is a **part of us**, all of us. Death happens as it is meant for your loved one and for each of us, whether we know the reason or not.

It is normal to feel sad. It is normal to feel numb. It is normal to feel lost. It is normal to feel empty. It is normal to feel angry. It is normal to feel *whatever* you are feeling.

All this time, you have been putting every ounce of your energy into caring for your loved one. As a result, you were likely suppressing as many emotions as possible. You may have felt the need to be strong and courageous. To do so, you hid and buried your true feelings to support your dying loved one in the best way possible.

Grief is experienced by each of us differently. In our own time, in our own way. Allow yourself this time just to **be**, noticing your feelings for what they are. Do not be afraid to seek personal or professional guidance and support. I encourage you to do so.

> *What I have learned is that grief is love that is lost. It is all the love you have to give. All the love that once had a place where it was welcomed with open arms. I now know grief is just love that is simply looking for a home.*

They say time heals all wounds, but losing someone you love just doesn't feel the same. And so, while that pain, sadness, emptiness, and heartache may never disappear, over time, you will learn *it* cannot control you. And, so, as consuming as it may feel, that grief will slowly begin to walk beside you.

Be gentle on yourself. Rest now. Move <u>slowly</u>.

Healing is, in itself, another journey.

PLEASE SHARE

If you found this book helpful in any way, big or small, I would greatly appreciate you leaving a review and providing feedback using the link below. I would be grateful for your advice to better serve our community.

Insert link below into your browser to leave a review!

https://www.amazon.com/review/create-review/?asin=B09GPZ3DT5

With the knowledge and information provided in this guidebook, I hope you will have peace in your mind and bring peace to your loved one's soul. I invite you to leave a review, share your thoughts, and let me know how else I may help you. If you believe this guidebook might help someone else, please share it with your friends, family, and community.

It important you know you are not alone in this. We have an entire community to support you. If you would like to hear more from me, I'd love to connect with you.

Join our Facebook Community Death.Care.Coach

Facebook Community Group: https://www.facebook.com/groups/death.care.coach

Instagram: @death.care.coach

Webpage (Under Construction): www.deathcarecoach.com

7
BONUS

"You will lose someone you can't live without, and your heart will be badly broken, and the bad news is that you never completely get over the loss of your beloved. But this is also the good news. They live forever in your broken heart that doesn't seal back up. And you come through. It's like having a broken leg that never heals perfectly – that still hurts when the weather gets cold, but you learn to dance with the limp"

— ANNE LAMOTT

Self-Care

This brief section explores the importance of **self-care**. Taking care of someone you love, especially at the end of their life, is a massive undertaking. Most of us will step into this caregiver role totally unprepared and without warning.

You will likely be so focused on providing care and comfort to your loved one that you will forget to take care of yourself. And this, my dear friends, is something you <u>must</u> prioritize.

You must **prioritize <u>your</u> health** so you can show up for your loved one. If you do not, you are not providing your loved one your absolute best.

Unfortunately, I have seen too many caregivers become absorbed tending to the needs of loved ones that their health also begins to fail. I, myself, have been guilty of this.

This self-neglect, this burnout, sneaks up on you without you noticing. So, for both your sake and for the sake of your loved one, be mindful. Act responsibly. Protect your needs. Because **self-care** is, in all respects, true **selflessness**.

Find time to **recharge** and refuel. Create your "me-time" schedule.

Brush your **teeth** every morning and every night.

<u>Feed</u> yourself breakfast, lunch, and dinner.

Stay **hydrated**. Keep a filled water bottle around at all times. Take small sips every hour.

Step <u>outside</u> of your house at least once a day.

Give yourself at least 7 hours of **sleep** per night.

Take at least 10 minutes every day to do something for <u>yourself</u>.

This could be a short walk. This could be closing your eyes and simply counting your breaths. This could be journaling. This could be listening to music. This could be reading a book.

What is one thing that will help you reconnect to your identity? What is one thing that brings you joy?

Do this. Every. Single. Day.

Reach out to your healthcare team to discuss various **resources** and options that may be available in your community or local health agencies to help you take the rest periods you need. Respite stays, adult day-care centers, and home health aide services are just a few of those options.

ACKNOWLEDGMENTS

There are too many people who have inspired me both personally and indirectly that led to the creation of this book to be able to thank individually.

To those who have allowed me to be with you during the most intimate, personal, vulnerable and yet most beautiful part of your life's journeys -- in other words, your dying journeys -- I thank you. You taught me what death and dying looks like and feels like in the physical, emotional, cultural, psychosocial, and spiritual realms. Your teachings have enabled me to further help those that have died after you, and those who will continue to die in the future. I thought of many of you and your stories while writing this book. You aren't here to see this now, but your death and dying journeys are impacting countless others.

To all the families and caregivers that have allowed me to act as a guide and a coach when the dying journeys of your loved ones presented the most challenging times of your lives, I thank you as well. You have shown me what true courage, strength, dedication, and love really means.

To my Granddad who reminded me of my life's calling to this service time and time again, especially in your final moments here with us. I always feel you in my heart. This book cover is your favorite place, my favorite place, and the place I know your spirit rests in peace.

To my sister, Sarah, who continues to inspire me in more ways than she knows, you have helped me break through fears I didn't even know existed. To my parents, thank you for unconditionally loving and supporting me, my dreams, and my passions. To Adam Holding, for helping make the creation of this book possible, for reproducing my photograph into this beautiful book cover, and for far more than I can describe here today. To my Uncle Bob, for guiding, editing, and helping me through so much of this process. To my cousin Danny, for coaching me through wandering visions and encouraging me every step of the way. To my cousin, Brooks, for graciously offering to help me record and edit this audiobook. To my friends, for keeping me accountable and encouraging my crazy dreams. To all those who are no longer part of my immediate life but inspired me to reach this moment. Each of you has impacted me in some way that has led me here today to share this information. I am utterly grateful for you all.

ABOUT THE AUTHOR

Katie Duncan, MSN, CRNP, AGPCNP-BC, is a national board-certified nurse practitioner, educator, author, and end-of-life care coach with a vision to rid society's stigma of death and dying.

She is a practicing adult-gerontology primary care nurse practitioner. She is also the founder and CEO of Death Care Coach, a company offering end-of-life expertise, consulting, education, and coaching to families, caregivers, and healthcare providers. Before founding Death Care Coach, she taught full-time as a Professor at Drexel University in the College of Nursing and Health Professions Undergraduate Program, and an adjunct Professor in the Nurse Practitioner Program.

Duncan has been working in healthcare for over 10 years in various roles and various specialties. She has spent time in hospital and intensive care settings. She has also worked in home-care and community settings, navigating her way into diverse homes while developing strong, trusting relationships with her patients and their families. In addition,

Duncan has spent time in sub-acute rehab, assisted living, independent living, nursing home, and long-term care facilities.

Of all the places Duncan has worked, her greatest love has always been end-of-life hospice care. It has been her honor to be at the bedside of irreplaceable fellow humans as they take their last breaths in their physical bodies.

Her journey has taught her that life is a precious gift, and there is an opportunity to find beauty even at the very end. As a result, Duncan has made it her mission to educate, coach, and provide holistic services focusing on end-of-life matters.

facebook.com/death.care.coach
instagram.com/death.care.coach
linkedin.com/in/k-duncan

THE CRUCIAL TOOLKIT FOR END-OF-LIFE CARE

Get Your Exclusive Copy Now!

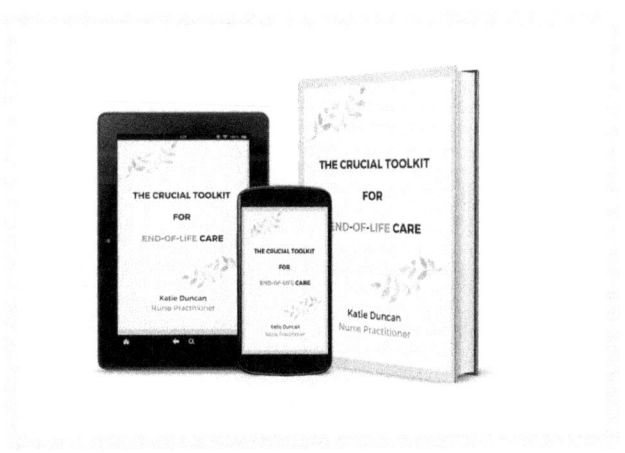

Insert the link below into your browser:
www.deathcarecoach.com

REFERENCES

11 Quotes From Harry Potter To Help You Cope With Loss. (2016). BuzzFeed. https://www.buzzfeed.com/rawaneewshah/the-bravest-man-i-ever-knew

82 Death Quotes that will Comfort and Inspire you. (2021). Sympathy Message Ideas. https://www.sympathymessageideas.com/death-quotes/

118th Annual Meeting of the American Association of Colleges of Pharmacy, Nashville, Tennessee, July 15-19, 2017. (2017). American Journal of Pharmaceutical Education, 81(5), 1.

American Family Physician. (2009). Care for People with a Severe or Complicated Illness. *American Family Physician, 79*(12). https://www.aafp.org/afp/2009/0615/p1059-s1.html

BHARADWAJ, P., MD, & Ward, K., MD. (2011). Palliative Sedation for a Patient with Terminal Illness. *American Family Physician, 83*(9), 1094–1095. https://www.aafp.org/afp/2011/0501/p1094.html

Blundon, E., Gallagher, R., & Ward, L. (2020). Electrophysiological evidence of preserved hearing at the end of life. *Scientific Reports.* Published. https://doi.org/10.1038/s41598-020-67234-9

Clary, P., MD, & Lawson, P., MD. (2009). Pharmacologic Pearls for End-of-Life Care. *American Family Physician, 79*(12), 1059–1065. https://www.aafp.org/afp/2009/0615/p1059.html

Committee on Approaching Death: Addressing Key End of Life Issues; Institute of Medicine. (2015). *Dying in America: Improving Quality and Honoring Individual Preferences Near the End of Life.* National Academies Press (US). https://pubmed.ncbi.nlm.nih.gov/25927121/

Committee on Approaching Death: Addressing Key End of Life Issues; Institute of Medicine. (2015). *Dying in America: Improving Quality and Honoring Individual Preferences Near the End of Life.* National Academies Press (US). https://www.ncbi.nlm.nih.gov/books/NBK285686/

Communication with Others as You Near the End of Life. (2019). American Cancer Society. https://www.cancer.org/treatment/end-of-life-care/nearing-the-end-of-life/communication.html

Corliss, J. (2019). *Six relaxation techniques to reduce stress.* Harvard Health Publishing. https://www.health.harvard.edu/mind-and-mood/six-relaxation-techniques-to-reduce-stress

Davis, M., MD. (2021). *Stopping nutrition and hydration at the end of life.* Uptodate. https://www.uptodate.com/contents/stopping-nutrition-and-hydration-at-the-end-of-life-search=end%20of%20life&topicRef=14241&source=see_link

Emotions and Coping as You Near the End of Life. (2019). American Cancer Society. https://www.cancer.org/treatment/end-of-life-care/nearing-the-end-of-life/emotions.html

Good Personal Hygiene. (n.d.). Arizona Department of Health Services. https://www.azdhs.gov/documents/preparedness/epidemiology-disease-control/disease-integrated-services/refugee-health/health-materials/english/english-personal-hygiene.pdf

Harman, S., MD, Bailey, F., MD, & Walling, A., MD, PhD. (2020). *Palliative care: The last hours and days of life.* Uptodate. https://www.uptodate.com/contents/palliative-care-the-last-hours-and-days-of-life?search=end%20of%20life&source=search_result&selectedTitle=1~150&usage_type=default&display_rank=1

Healthy Transfers. (2019). National Caregivers Library. http://www.caregiverslibrary.org/Caregivers-Resources/GRP-Home-Care/HSGRP-Personal-Care-Activities/Healthy-Transfers-Article

Helen Keller > Quotes > Quotable Quote. (n.d.). Goodreads. https://www.goodreads.com/quotes/4202-what-we-once-enjoyed-and-deeply-loved-we-can-never

Hill, N. (1937). *Think and Grow Rich.* The Ralston Society.

Hospice Foundation of America. (n.d.). *Signs of Approaching Death.* https://hospicefoundation.org/Hospice-Care/Signs-of-Approaching-Death

Hospice Foundation of America. (2011). *A Caregiver's Guide to the Dying Process.* https://hospicefoundation.org/hfa/media/Files/Hospice_TheDyingProcess_Docutech-READERSPREADS.pdf

J.K. Rowling > Quotes > Quotable Quote. (n.d.). Goodreads. https://www.goodreads.com/quotes/4864-to-the-well-organized-mind-death-is-but-the-next-great

Kolb, H., Snowden, A., & Stevens, E. (2018). Systematic review and narrative summary: Treatments for and risk factors associated with respiratory tract secretions (death rattle) in the dying adult. *Journal of Advanced Nursing, 74*(7). https://doi.org/10.1111/jan.13557

Leach C. (2019). Nausea and vomiting in palliative care. *Clinical medicine (London, England), 19*(4), 299–301. https://doi.org/10.7861/clinmedicine.19-4-299

Meier, D., MD, FACP, McCormick, E., MD, & Lagman, R., MD, MPH, FACP, FAAHPM. (2020). *Hospice: Philosophy of care and appropriate utilization in the United States.* Uptodate.

https://www.uptodate.com/contents/hospice-philosophy-of-care-and-appropriate-utilization-in-the-united-states?search=end%20of%20life&topicRef=14241&source=see_link

Oxygen safety. (2021). MedlinePlus. https://medlineplus.gov/ency/patientinstructions/000049.htm

Persson, H., Sandgren, A., Fürst, C., Ahlström, G., & Behm, L. (2018). Early and late signs that precede dying among older persons in nursing homes: the multidisciplinary team's perspective. *BMC Geriatrics, 18*(134). https://bmcgeriatr.biomedcentral.com/articles/10.1186/s12877-018-0825-0#citeas

Physical Changes as You Near the End of Life. (2019). American Cancer Society. https://www.cancer.org/treatment/end-of-life-care/nearing-the-end-of-life/physical-symptoms.html

Providing Care and Comfort at the End of Life. (n.d.). National Institute on Aging. https://www.nia.nih.gov/health/providing-comfort-end-life

Rome, R., MSN, FNP-C., Luminais, H., RN, Bourgeois, D., MN, APRN, ACNS-BC, & Blais, C., MD, MPH, FACP, FAAHPM. (2011). The Role of Palliative Care at the End of Life. *The Ochsner Journal, 11*(4), 348–352. https://www.ncbi.nlm.nih.gov/pmc/articles/PMC3241069/

Ross, A., MD, PhD. (2017). End-of-Life Care: Managing Common Symptoms. *American Family Physician, 95*(6), 356–351. https://www.aafp.org/afp/2017/0315/p356.html

Ross, D., M. D. ,. Ph. D., & Alexander, C., M. D. (2001). Management of Common Symptoms in Terminally Ill Patients: Part I. Fatigue, Anorexia, Cachexia, Nausea and Vomiting. *American Family Physician, 64*(5), 807–815. https://www.aafp.org/afp/2001/0901/p807.html

Saying Goodbye. (2019). American Cancer Society. https://www.cancer.org/treatment/end-of-life-care/nearing-the-end-of-life/saying-goodbye.html

Signs of Approaching Death. (2018). Hospice Foundation of America. https://hospicefoundation.org/Hospice-Care/Signs-of-Approaching-Death

Stanford Health Care. (n.d.). *Management of Pain Without Medications.* https://stanfordhealthcare.org/medical-conditions/pain/pain/treatments/non-pharmacological-pain-management.html

Steve Jobs > Quotes > Quotable Quote. (n.d.). Goodreads. https://www.goodreads.com/quotes/427423-no-one-wants-to-die-even-people-who-want-to

Taylor, A., *& Box, M. (1999). Multicultural Palliative Care Guidelines. Palliative Care Council of South Australia.* https://palliativecare.org.au/wp-content/uploads/2015/05/Multicultural-palliative-care-guidelines.pdf

What is the best approach to decreasing respiratory secretions at the end of life? (2021). Canadian Virtual Hospice. https://www.virtualhospice.ca/en_US/Main+Site+Navigation/Home/For+Professionals/For+Professionals/Quick+Consults/Symptoms/What+is+the+best+approach+to+decreasing+respiratory+secretions+at+the+end+of+life_.aspx

What to Do When a Loved One Dies. (2020). AARP. https://www.aarp.org/home-family/friends-family/info-2020/when-loved-one-dies-checklist.html

What to Expect When a Person With Cancer is Nearing Death. (2019). American Cancer Society. https://www.cancer.org/treatment/end-of-life-care/nearing-the-end-of-life/death.html

"You've got to find what you love," Jobs says. (2005). Stanford News. https://news.stanford.edu/2005/06/14/jobs-061505/